MW01115284

Global Strategy for Infant and Young Child Feeding

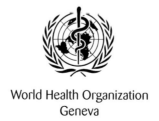

World Health Organization
Geneva

WHO Library Cataloguing-in-Publication Data

Global strategy for infant and young child feeding.

1.Infant nutrition 2.Breast feeding 3.Feeding behavior 4.National health programs
5.Health policy 6.Guidelines I.World Health Organization
II. UNICEF

ISBN 92 4 156221 8   (NLM classification: WS 120)

Designed by minimum graphics
Printed in Singapore

Contents

Abbreviations

FAO	Food and Agriculture Organization of the United Nations
HIV/AIDS	Human immunodeficiency virus/acquired immunodeficiency syndrome
ILO	International Labour Organization
UNAIDS	Joint United Nations Programme on HIV/AIDS
UNFPA	United Nations Population Fund
UNHCR	United Nations High Commission for Refugees
UNICEF	United Nations Children's Fund
WHO	World Health Organization

Foreword

WHO and UNICEF jointly developed the Global Strategy for Infant and Young Child Feeding to revitalize world attention to the impact that feeding practices have on the nutritional status, growth and development, health, and thus the very survival of infants and young children.

The Global Strategy is based on the evidence of nutrition's significance in the early months and years of life, and of the crucial role that appropriate feeding practices play in achieving optimal health outcomes. Lack of breastfeeding – and especially lack of exclusive breastfeeding during the first half-year of life – are important risk factors for infant and childhood morbidity and mortality that are only compounded by inappropriate complementary feeding. The life-long impact includes poor school performance, reduced productivity, and impaired intellectual and social development.

The Strategy is the result of a comprehensive two-year participatory process. The aim, from the outset, was to move towards formulating a sound approach to alleviating the tragic burden borne by the world's children – 50 to 70% of the burden of diarrhoeal disease, measles, malaria and lower respiratory infections in childhood are attributable to undernutrition – and to contribute to a lasting reduction in poverty and deprivation.

This exercise provided an exceptional opportunity to re-examine critically, in the light of the latest scientific and epidemiological evidence, the fundamental factors affecting feeding practices for infants and young children. At the same time, it renewed commitment to continuing joint action consistent with the Baby-friendly Hospital Initiative, the International Code of Marketing of Breast-milk Substitutes, and the Innocenti Declaration on the Protection, Promotion and Support of Breast-feeding.

The Strategy is intended as a *guide for action*; it identifies interventions with a proven positive impact, it emphasizes providing mothers and families the support they need to carry out their crucial roles, and it explicitly defines the obligations and responsibilities in this regard of governments, international organizations and other concerned parties.

We are proud of the unanimous endorsement that the governing bodies of our two agencies have pronounced in support of the Global Strategy.[1] The first necessary political step has been taken. It is now time for everyone concerned – governments as well as all the other innumerable actors throughout society – to move swiftly and deliberately to give tangible effect to the Strategy's vital aim and practical objectives. There can be no delay in applying the accumulated knowledge and experience to help make our world a truly fit environment where *all* children can thrive and achieve their full potential.

Gro Harlem Brundtland
  MD, MPH
Director-General
World Health Organization

Carol Bellamy
Executive Director
United Nations Children's
  Fund

---

[1] The Global Strategy was endorsed, by consensus, on 18 May 2002 by the Fifty-fifth World Health Assembly, and on 16 September 2002 by the UNICEF Executive Board (see annex).

1. Introduction

The Executive Board of the World Health Organization, at its 101st session in January 1998, called for a revitalization of the global commitment to appropriate infant and young child nutrition, and in particular breastfeeding and complementary feeding. Subsequently, in close collaboration with the United Nations Children's Fund, WHO organized a consultation (Geneva, 13–17 March 2000) to assess infant and young child feeding practices, review key interventions, and formulate a comprehensive strategy for the next decade.

Following discussions at the Fifty-third World Health Assembly in May 2000 and the 107th session of the Executive Board in January 2001 of the outline and critical issues of the global strategy, the Fifty-fourth World Health Assembly (May 2001) reviewed progress and requested the Director-General to submit the strategy to the Executive Board at its 109th session and to the Fifty-fifth World Health Assembly, respectively in January and May 2002.[1]

During their discussion of the draft of the global strategy, members of the Executive Board commended the setting in motion of the consultative, science-based process that had led to its formulation as a guide for developing country-specific approaches to improving feeding practices. They also welcomed the strategy's integrated and comprehensive approach. Several members made suggestions with regard to the exact wording of the draft strategy. These suggestions were taken carefully into account in preparing the strategy, as were comments from Member States following the Board's 109th session[2] and observations of other interested parties, including professional associations, nongovernmental organizations and the processed-food industry. Stressing the validity of a well-structured draft, the Executive Board recommended that the Health Assembly endorse the global strategy and that Member States

---

[1] Resolution WHA54.2, paragraph 3(6).
[2] Provided in response to circular letter C.L.5.2002, dated 8 February 2002.

implement it, as appropriate to national circumstances, in order to promote optimal feeding for all infants and young children.[1]

An emerging policy framework

From the outset it was agreed that the global strategy should build on past and continuing achievements – particularly the Baby-friendly Hospital Initiative (1991), the International Code of Marketing of Breast-milk Substitutes (1981) and the Innocenti Declaration on the Protection, Promotion and Support of Breastfeeding (1990) – in the overall context of national policies and programmes on nutrition and child health, and consistent with the World Declaration and Plan of Action for Nutrition.[2] However, it should go further and emphasize the need for comprehensive national policies on infant and young child feeding, including guidelines on ensuring appropriate feeding of infants and young children in exceptionally difficult circumstances, and the need to ensure that all health services protect, promote and support exclusive breastfeeding and timely and adequate complementary feeding with continued breastfeeding.

Two principles guided the development of the strategy: it should be grounded on the best available scientific and epidemiological evidence, and it should be as participatory as possible. Consequently, the work involved extensive review of the scientific literature and several technical consultations. The latter focused on both crucial elements of the strategy and specific issues. For instance, the WHO/UNICEF consultation in March 2000 brought together experts in strategic and programmatic aspects of the subject and representatives of ILO, UNHCR and UNAIDS; the UNAIDS/UNICEF/UNFPA/WHO Interagency Task Team meeting (Geneva, 11–13 October 2000) considered the prevention of mother-to-child transmission of HIV;[3] and the expert consulta-

---

[1] Resolution EB109.R18.

[2] *World Declaration and Plan of Action for Nutrition.* International Conference on Nutrition, Rome, FAO/WHO, 1992.

[3] New data on the prevention of mother-to-child transmission of HIV and their policy implications: conclusions and recommendations. WHO technical consultation on behalf of the UNFPA/UNICEF/WHO/UNAIDS Interagency Task Team on Mother-to-Child Transmission of HIV, October 2001, Geneva, WHO (document WHO/RHR/01.28).

tion (Geneva, 28–30 March 2001) reviewed the optimal duration of exclusive breastfeeding.[1]

Consistent with an approach in which countries participated, from the outset, in tailoring the strategy to their specific needs, during the period 2000–2001 the draft strategy was considered at country consultations in Brazil, China, Philippines, Scotland, Sri Lanka, Thailand and Zimbabwe. Six regional consultations followed with representatives of more than 100 Member States and the participation of UNICEF, FAO, ILO, the International Lactation Consultant Association, the International Baby Food Action Network, and the World Alliance for Breastfeeding Action. On the basis of the inputs provided and the principles that evolved through this process, the following policy framework emerged.

- Inappropriate feeding practices and their consequences are major obstacles to sustainable socioeconomic development and poverty reduction. Governments will be unsuccessful in their efforts to accelerate economic development in any significant long-term sense until optimal child growth and development, especially through appropriate feeding practices, are ensured.

- Appropriate evidence-based feeding practices are essential for attaining and maintaining proper nutrition and health.

- Mothers and babies form an inseparable biological and social unit; the health and nutrition of one group cannot be divorced from the health and nutrition of the other.

- Keeping improved infant and young child feeding high on the public health agenda is crucial to consolidating gains made during the past two decades.

- Twenty years after adoption of the International Code of Marketing of Breast-milk Substitutes and 10 years into giving practical effect to the World Declaration and Plan of Action for Nutrition, the Innocenti Declaration and the Baby-friendly Hospital Initiative, it is time for governments, the international community and other concerned parties to renew their commit-

[1] The optimal duration of exclusive breastfeeding. Report of an expert consultation. Geneva, WHO (document WHO/NHD/01.09, WHO/FCH/CAH/01.24) March 2001.

ment to promoting the health and nutrition of infants and young children and to work together for this purpose.

- Although not every component is new, what is novel about the global strategy is its *integrated comprehensive approach* and the *degree of urgency* called for in implementing it, in order to deal effectively with so elementary a challenge as ensuring appropriate feeding for the world's children.

- The most rational and economical approach to achieving the strategy's aim and objectives is to use *existing* health and intersectoral structures, reinforced where necessary.

- Success in implementing the global strategy rests, first and foremost, on achieving political commitment at the highest level and assembling the indispensable human and financial resources.

- Additional high-priority conditions for success include definition of suitable goals and objectives, a realistic timeline for their achievement, and measurable process and output indicators that will permit an accurate monitoring and evaluation of action taken and a rapid response to identified needs.

2. Global strategy for infant and young child feeding

Defining the challenge

1. Malnutrition has been responsible, directly or indirectly, for 60% of the 10.9 million deaths annually among children under five. Well over two-thirds of these deaths, which are often associated with inappropriate feeding practices, occur during the first year of life. No more than 35% of infants worldwide are exclusively breastfed during the first four months of life; complementary feeding frequently begins too early or too late, and foods are often nutritionally inadequate and unsafe. Malnourished children who survive are more frequently sick and suffer the life-long consequences of impaired development. Rising incidences of overweight and obesity in children are also a matter of serious concern. Because poor feeding practices are a major threat to social and economic development, they are among the most serious obstacles to attaining and maintaining health that face this age group.

2. The health and nutritional status of mothers and children are intimately linked. Improved infant and young child feeding begins with ensuring the health and nutritional status of women, in their own right, throughout all stages of life and continues with women as providers for their children and families. Mothers and infants form a biological and social unit; they also share problems of malnutrition and ill-health. Whatever is done to solve these problems concerns both mothers and children together.

3. The global strategy for infant and young child feeding is based on respect, protection, facilitation and fulfilment of accepted human rights principles. Nutrition is a crucial, universally recognized component of the child's right to the enjoyment of the highest attainable standard of health as stated in the Convention on the Rights of the Child. Children have the right to adequate nutrition and access to safe and nutritious food, and both are essential for fulfilling their right to the highest attainable standard of health. Women, in turn,

have the right to proper nutrition, to decide how to feed their children, and to full information and appropriate conditions that will enable them to carry out their decisions. These rights are not yet realized in many environments.

4. Rapid social and economic change only intensifies the difficulties that families face in properly feeding and caring for their children. Expanding urbanization results in more families that depend on informal or intermittent employment with uncertain incomes and few or no maternity benefits. Both self-employed and nominally employed rural women face heavy workloads, usually with no maternity protection. Meanwhile, traditional family and community support structures are being eroded, resources devoted to supporting health- and, especially, nutrition-related, services are dwindling, accurate information on optimal feeding practices is lacking, and the number of food-insecure rural and urban households is on the rise.

5. The HIV pandemic and the risk of mother-to-child transmission of HIV through breastfeeding pose unique challenges to the promotion of breastfeeding, even among unaffected families. Complex emergencies, which are often characterized by population displacement, food insecurity and armed conflict, are increasing in number and intensity, further compromising the care and feeding of infants and young children the world over. Refugees and internally displaced persons alone currently number more than 40 million, including 5.5 million under-five children.

Determining the aim and objectives

6. The *aim* of this strategy is to improve – through optimal feeding – the nutritional status, growth and development, health, and thus the survival of infants and young children.

7. The strategy's specific *objectives* are:

- to raise awareness of the main problems affecting infant and young child feeding, identify approaches to their solution, and provide a framework of essential interventions;

- to increase the commitment of governments, international

organizations and other concerned parties[1] for optimal feeding practices for infants and young children;

- to create an environment that will enable mothers, families and other caregivers in all circumstances to make – and implement – informed choices about optimal feeding practices for infants and young children.

8. The strategy is intended as a guide for action; it is based on accumulated evidence of the significance of the early months and years of life for child growth and development and it identifies interventions with a proven positive impact during this period. Moreover to remain dynamic, successful strategy implementation will rely on keeping pace with developments, while new clinical and population-based research is stimulated and behavioural concerns are investigated.

9. No single intervention or group can succeed in meeting the challenge; implementing the strategy thus calls for increased political will, public investment, awareness among health workers, involvement of families and communities, and collaboration between governments, international organizations and other concerned parties that will ultimately ensure that all necessary action is taken.

Promoting appropriate feeding for infants and young children

10. *Breastfeeding* is an unequalled way of providing ideal food for the healthy growth and development of infants; it is also an integral part of the reproductive process with important implications for the health of mothers. As a global public health recommendation, infants should be exclusively breastfed for the first six months of

---

[1] For the purposes of this strategy, other concerned parties include professional bodies, training institutions, industrial and commercial enterprises and their associations, nongovernmental organizations whether or not formally registered, religious and charitable organizations and citizens' associations such as community-based breastfeeding support networks and consumer groups.

life to achieve optimal growth, development and health.[1] Thereafter, to meet their evolving nutritional requirements, infants should receive nutritionally adequate and safe complementary foods while breastfeeding continues for up to two years of age or beyond. Exclusive breastfeeding from birth is possible except for a few medical conditions, and unrestricted exclusive breastfeeding results in ample milk production.

11. Even though it is a natural act, breastfeeding is also a learned behaviour. Virtually all mothers can breastfeed provided they have accurate information, and support within their families and communities and from the health care system. They should also have access to skilled practical help from, for example, trained health workers, lay and peer counsellors, and certified lactation consultants, who can help to build mothers' confidence, improve feeding technique, and prevent or resolve breastfeeding problems.

12. Women in paid employment can be helped to continue breastfeeding by being provided with minimum enabling conditions, for example paid maternity leave, part-time work arrangements, on-site crèches, facilities for expressing and storing breast milk, and breastfeeding breaks (see paragraph 28).

13. Infants are particularly vulnerable during the transition period when *complementary feeding* begins. Ensuring that their nutritional needs are met thus requires that complementary foods be:

- *timely* – meaning that they are introduced when the need for energy and nutrients exceeds what can be provided through exclusive and frequent breastfeeding;

- *adequate* – meaning that they provide sufficient energy, protein and micronutrients to meet a growing child's nutritional needs;

- *safe* – meaning that they are hygienically stored and prepared, and fed with clean hands using clean utensils and not bottles and teats;

---

[1] As formulated in the conclusions and recommendations of the expert consultation (Geneva, 28–30 March 2001) that completed the systematic review of the optimal duration of exclusive breastfeeding (see document A54/INF.DOC./4). See also resolution WHA54.2.

8

- *properly fed* – meaning that they are given consistent with a child's signals of appetite and satiety, and that meal frequency and feeding method – actively encouraging the child, even during illness, to consume sufficient food using fingers, spoon or self-feeding – are suitable for age.

14. Appropriate complementary feeding depends on accurate *information* and skilled support from the family, community and health care system. Inadequate knowledge about appropriate foods and feeding practices is often a greater determinant of malnutrition than the lack of food. Moreover, diversified approaches are required to ensure access to foods that will adequately meet energy and nutrient needs of growing children, for example use of home- and community-based technologies to enhance nutrient density, bioavailability and the micronutrient content of local foods.

15. Providing sound and culture-specific nutrition counselling to mothers of young children and recommending the widest possible use of indigenous foodstuffs will help ensure that *local foods* are prepared and fed safely in the home. The agriculture sector has a particularly important role to play in ensuring that suitable foods for use in complementary feeding are produced, readily available and affordable.

16. In addition, *low-cost complementary foods*, prepared with locally available ingredients using suitable small-scale production technologies in community settings, can help to meet the nutritional needs of older infants and young children. *Industrially processed complementary foods* also provide an option for some mothers who have the means to buy them and the knowledge and facilities to prepare and feed them safely. Processed-food products for infants and young children should, when sold or otherwise distributed, meet applicable standards recommended by the Codex Alimentarius Commission and also the Codex Code of Hygienic Practice for Foods for Infants and Children.

17. *Food fortification* and universal or targeted *nutrient supplementation* may also help to ensure that older infants and young children receive adequate amounts of micronutrients.

Exercising other feeding options

18. The vast majority of mothers can and should breastfeed, just as the vast majority of infants can and should be breastfed. Only under exceptional circumstances can a mother's milk be considered unsuitable for her infant. For those few health situations where infants cannot, or should not, be breastfed, the choice of the best alternative – expressed breast milk from an infant's own mother, breast milk from a healthy wet-nurse or a human-milk bank, or a breast-milk substitute fed with a cup, which is a safer method than a feeding bottle and teat – depends on individual circumstances.

19. For infants who do not receive breast milk, feeding with a suitable breast-milk substitute – for example an infant formula prepared in accordance with applicable Codex Alimentarius standards, or a home-prepared formula with micronutrient supplements – should be demonstrated only by health workers, or other community workers if necessary, and only to the mothers and other family members who need to use it; and the information given should include adequate instructions for appropriate preparation and the health hazards of inappropriate preparation and use. Infants who are not breastfed, for whatever reason, should receive special attention from the health and social welfare system since they constitute a risk group.

Feeding in exceptionally difficult circumstances

20. Families in *difficult situations* require special attention and practical support to be able to feed their children adequately. In such cases the likelihood of not breastfeeding increases, as do the dangers of artificial feeding and inappropriate complementary feeding. Wherever possible, mothers and babies should remain together and be provided the support they need to exercise the most appropriate feeding option under the circumstances.

21. Infants and young children who are *malnourished* are most often found in environments where improving the quality and quantity of food intake is particularly problematic. To prevent a recurrence and to overcome the effects of chronic malnutrition, these children need extra attention both during the early rehabilitation phase and over the longer term. Nutritionally adequate and safe complemen-

tary foods may be particularly difficult to obtain and dietary supplements may be required for these children. Continued frequent
breastfeeding and, when necessary, relactation are important pre-
ventive steps since malnutrition often has its origin in inadequate
or disrupted breastfeeding.

22. The proportion of infants with *low birth weight* varies from 6% to
more than 28% depending on the setting. Most are born at or near
term and can breastfeed within the first hour after birth. Breast
milk is particularly important for preterm infants and the small
proportion of term infants with very low birth weight; they are at
increased risk of infection, long-term ill-health and death.

23. Infants and children are among the most vulnerable victims of natural or human-induced *emergencies*. Interrupted breastfeeding and
inappropriate complementary feeding heighten the risk of malnutrition, illness and mortality. Uncontrolled distribution of breast-
milk substitutes, for example in refugee settings, can lead to early
and unnecessary cessation of breastfeeding. For the vast majority
of infants emphasis should be on protecting, promoting and supporting breastfeeding and ensuring timely, safe and appropriate
complementary feeding. There will always be a small number of
infants who have to be fed on breast-milk substitutes. Suitable substitutes, procured, distributed and fed safely as part of the regular
inventory of foods and medicines, should be provided.

24. An estimated 1.6 million children are born to *HIV-infected women*
each year, mainly in low-income countries. The absolute risk of HIV
transmission through breastfeeding for more than one year – glo-
bally between 10% and 20% – needs to be balanced against the
increased risk of morbidity and mortality when infants are not
breastfed. All HIV-infected mothers should receive counselling,
which includes provision of general information about meeting their
own nutritional requirements and about the risks and benefits of
various feeding options, and specific guidance in selecting the option most likely to be suitable for their situation. Adequate *replacement feeding* is needed for infants born to HIV-positive mothers who
choose not to breastfeed. It requires a suitable breast-milk substitute, for example an infant formula prepared in accordance with
applicable Codex Alimentarius standards, or a home-prepared formula with micronutrient supplements. Heat-treated breast milk, or

breast milk provided by an HIV-negative donor mother, may be an option in some cases. To reduce the risk of interfering with the promotion of breastfeeding for the great majority, providing a breast-milk substitute for these infants should be consistent with the principles and aim of the International Code of Marketing of Breast-milk Substitutes (see paragraph 19). For mothers who test negative for HIV, or who are untested, exclusive breastfeeding remains the recommended feeding option (see paragraph 10).

25. Children living in *special circumstances* also require extra attention – for example, orphans and children in foster care, and children born to adolescent mothers, mothers suffering from physical or mental disabilities, drug- or alcohol-dependence, or mothers who are imprisoned or part of disadvantaged or otherwise marginalized populations.

Improving feeding practices

26. Mothers, fathers and other caregivers should have access to objective, consistent and complete *information* about appropriate feeding practices, free from commercial influence. In particular, they need to know about the recommended period of exclusive and continued breastfeeding; the timing of the introduction of complementary foods; what types of food to give, how much and how often; and how to feed these foods safely.

27. Mothers should have access to *skilled support* to help them initiate and sustain appropriate feeding practices, and to prevent difficulties and overcome them when they occur. Knowledgeable health workers are well placed to provide this support, which should be a routine part not only of regular prenatal, delivery and postnatal care but also of services provided for the well baby and sick child. Community-based networks offering mother-to-mother support, and trained breastfeeding counsellors working within, or closely with, the health care system, also have an important role to play in this regard. Where fathers are concerned, research shows that breastfeeding is enhanced by the support and companionship they provide as family providers and caregivers.

28. Mothers should also be able to continue breastfeeding and caring for their children after they return to *paid employment*. This can be accomplished by implementing maternity protection legislation and related measures consistent with ILO Maternity Protection Convention, 2000 No. 183 and Maternity Protection Recommendation, 2000 No. 191. Maternity leave, day-care facilities and paid breastfeeding breaks should be available for all women employed outside the home.

29. Continuing clinical and population-based *research* and investigation of behavioural concerns are essential ingredients for improving feeding practices. Crucial areas include completion and application of the new international growth reference, prevention and control of micronutrient malnutrition, programmatic approaches and community-based interventions for improving breastfeeding and complementary feeding practices, improving maternal nutritional status and pregnancy outcome, and interventions for preventing mother-to-child transmission of HIV in relation to infant feeding.

Achieving the strategy's objectives

30. A first step to achieving the objectives of this strategy is to reaffirm the relevance – indeed the urgency – of the four operational targets of the Innocenti Declaration on the Protection, Promotion and Support of Breastfeeding:[1]

- appointing a national breastfeeding coordinator with appropriate authority, and establishing a multisectoral national breastfeeding committee composed of representatives from relevant government departments, nongovernmental organizations, and health professional associations;

- ensuring that every facility providing maternity services fully practices all the "Ten steps to successful breastfeeding" set out in the

---

[1] Meeting in Florence, Italy, in July 1990, government policy-makers from more than 30 countries adopted the Innocenti Declaration. The Forty-fourth World Health Assembly, in 1991, welcomed the Declaration as "a basis for international health policy and action" and requested the Director-General to monitor achievement of its targets (resolution WHA44.33).

WHO/UNICEF statement on breastfeeding and maternity services;[1]

- giving effect to the principles and aim of the International Code of Marketing of Breast-milk Substitutes and subsequent relevant Health Assembly resolutions in their entirety;

- enacting imaginative legislation protecting the breastfeeding rights of working women and establishing means for its enforcement.

31. Many governments have taken important steps towards realizing these targets and much has been achieved as a result, notably through the Baby-friendly Hospital Initiative and the legislation and other measures that have been adopted with regard to the marketing of breast-milk substitutes. Achievements are far from uniform, however, and there are signs of weakened commitment, for example in the face of the HIV/AIDS pandemic and the number and gravity of complex emergencies affecting infants and young children. Moreover, the Innocenti Declaration focuses uniquely on breastfeeding. Thus, additional targets are needed to reflect a comprehensive approach to meeting care and feeding requirements during the first three years of life through a wide range of interrelated actions.

32. In the light of accumulated scientific evidence, and policy and programme experience, the time is right for governments, with the support of international organizations and other concerned parties:

- to reconsider how best to ensure the appropriate feeding of infants and young children and to renew their collective commitment to meeting this challenge;

- to constitute effective broad-based bodies to lead the implementation of this strategy as a coordinated multisectoral national response by all concerned parties to the multiple challenges of infant and young child feeding;[2] and

---

[1] *Protecting, promoting and supporting breastfeeding: the special role of maternity services.* A joint WHO/UNICEF statement. Geneva, WHO, 1989.

[2] Consistent with the first target of the Innocenti Declaration, more than 100 countries have already appointed a national breastfeeding coordinator and established a multisectoral national committee. These arrangements could form the basis for the creation of the new body called for here.

- to establish a system to monitor regularly feeding practices, assess trends using sex-disaggregated data and evaluate the impact of interventions.

33. With these considerations in mind, the global strategy includes as a priority for all governments the achievement of the following additional operational targets:[1]

- to develop, implement, monitor and evaluate a comprehensive policy on infant and young child feeding, in the context of national policies and programmes for nutrition, child and reproductive health, and poverty reduction;

- to ensure that the health and other relevant sectors protect, promote and support exclusive breastfeeding for six months and continued breastfeeding up to two years of age or beyond, while providing women access to the support they require – in the family, community and workplace – to achieve this goal;

- to promote timely, adequate, safe and appropriate complementary feeding with continued breastfeeding;

- to provide guidance on feeding infants and young children in exceptionally difficult circumstances, and on the related support required by mothers, families and other caregivers;

- to consider what new legislation or other suitable measures may be required, as part of a comprehensive policy on infant and young child feeding, to give effect to the principles and aim of the International Code of Marketing of Breast-milk Substitutes and to subsequent relevant Health Assembly resolutions.

Implementing high-priority action

34. A comprehensive national policy, based on a thorough needs assessment, should foster an environment that protects, promotes and supports appropriate infant and young child feeding practices. An effective feeding policy consistent with efforts to promote overall household food security requires the following critical interventions:

---

[1] Governments should set a realistic date for achievement of all the global strategy's targets and define measurable indicators to assess their progress in this regard.

For protection

- adopting and monitoring application of a policy of maternity entitlements, consistent with the ILO Maternity Protection Convention and Recommendation, in order to facilitate breastfeeding by women in paid employment, including those whom the standards describe as engaging in atypical forms of dependent work, for example part-time, domestic and intermittent employment;

- ensuring that processed complementary foods are marketed for use at an appropriate age, and that they are safe, culturally acceptable, affordable and nutritionally adequate, in accordance with relevant Codex Alimentarius standards;

- implementing and monitoring existing measures to give effect to the International Code of Marketing of Breast-milk Substitutes and to subsequent relevant Health Assembly resolutions, and, where appropriate, strengthening them or adopting new measures;

For promotion

- ensuring that all who are responsible for communicating with the general public, including educational and media authorities, provide accurate and complete information about appropriate infant and young child feeding practices, taking into account prevailing social, cultural and environmental circumstances;

For support through the health care system

- providing skilled counselling and help for infant and young child feeding, for instance at well-baby clinics, during immunization sessions, and in in- and out-patient services for sick children, nutrition services, and reproductive health and maternity services;

- ensuring that hospital routines and procedures remain fully supportive of the successful initiation and establishment of breastfeeding through implementation of the Baby-friendly Hospital Initiative, monitoring and reassessing already designated facilities, and expanding the Initiative to include clinics, health centres and paediatric hospitals;

- increasing access to antenatal care and education about breast-feeding, to delivery practices which support breastfeeding and to follow-up care which helps to ensure continued breastfeeding;

- promoting good nutrition for pregnant and lactating women;

- monitoring the growth and development of infants and young children as a routine nutrition intervention, with particular attention to low-birth-weight and sick infants and those born to HIV-positive mothers, and ensuring that mothers and families receive appropriate counselling;

- providing guidance on appropriate complementary feeding with emphasis on the use of suitable locally available foods which are prepared and fed safely;

- promoting adequate intake of essential nutrients through access to suitable – including fortified – local foods and, when necessary, micronutrient supplements;

- enabling mothers to remain with their hospitalized children to ensure continued breastfeeding and adequate complementary feeding and, where feasible, allow breastfed children to stay with their hospitalized mothers;

- ensuring effective therapeutic feeding of sick and malnourished children, including the provision of skilled breastfeeding support when required;

- training health workers who care for mothers, children and families with regard to:

  — counselling and assistance skills needed for breastfeeding, complementary feeding, HIV and infant feeding and, when necessary, feeding with a breast-milk substitute,

  — feeding during illness,

  — health workers' responsibilities under the International Code of Marketing of Breast-milk Substitutes;

- revising and reforming pre-service curricula for all health workers, nutritionists and allied professionals to provide appropriate information and advice on infant and young child feeding for use by families and those involved in the field of infant and young child nutrition;

17

For support in the community

- promoting development of community-based support networks to help ensure appropriate infant and young child feeding, for example mother-to-mother support groups and peer or lay counsellors, to which hospitals and clinics can refer mothers on discharge;

- ensuring that community-based support networks not only are welcome within the health care system but also participate actively in the planning and provision of services;

For support for feeding infants and young children in exceptionally difficult circumstances

- ensuring that health workers have accurate and up-to-date information about infant feeding policies and practices, and that they have the specific knowledge and skills required to support caregivers and children in all aspects of infant and young child feeding in exceptionally difficult circumstances;

- creating conditions that will facilitate exclusive breastfeeding, by provision, for example, of appropriate maternity care, extra food rations and drinking-water for pregnant and lactating women, and staff who have breastfeeding counselling skills;

- ensuring that suitable – preferably locally available – complementary foods are selected and fed, consistent with the age and nutritional needs of older infants and young children;

- searching actively for malnourished infants and young children so that their condition can be identified and treated, they can be appropriately fed, and their caregivers can be supported;

- giving guidance for identifying infants who have to be fed on breast-milk substitutes, ensuring that a suitable substitute is provided and fed safely for as long as needed by the infants concerned, and preventing any "spillover effect" of artificial feeding into the general population;

- ensuring that health workers with knowledge and experience in all aspects of breastfeeding and replacement feeding are available to counsel HIV-positive women;

- adapting the Baby-friendly Hospital Initiative by taking account of HIV/AIDS and by ensuring that those responsible for emergency preparedness are well trained to support appropriate feeding practices consistent with the Initiative's universal principles;

- ensuring that whenever breast-milk substitutes are required for social or medical reasons, for example for orphans or in the case of HIV-positive mothers, they are provided for as long as the infants concerned need them.

Obligations and responsibilities

35. Governments, international organizations and other concerned parties share responsibility for ensuring the fulfilment of the right of children to the highest attainable standard of health and the right of women to full and unbiased information, and adequate health care and nutrition. Each partner should acknowledge and embrace its responsibilities for improving the feeding of infants and young children and for mobilizing required resources. All partners should work together to achieve fully this strategy's aim and objectives, including by forming fully transparent innovative alliances and partnerships consistent with accepted principles for avoiding conflict of interest.

Governments

36. The primary obligation of governments is to formulate, implement, monitor and evaluate a comprehensive *national policy* on infant and young child feeding. In addition to political commitment at the highest level, a successful policy depends on effective national co-ordination to ensure full collaboration of all concerned government agencies, international organizations and other concerned parties. This implies continual collection and evaluation of relevant information on feeding policies and practices. Regional and local governments also have an important role to play in implementing this strategy.

37. A detailed *action plan* should accompany the comprehensive policy, including defined goals and objectives, a timeline for their achievement, allocation of responsibilities for the plan's implementation

and measurable indicators for its monitoring and evaluation. For this purpose, governments should seek, when appropriate, the co-operation of appropriate international organizations and other agencies, including global and regional lending institutions. The plan should be compatible with, and form an integral part of, all other activities designed to contribute to optimal infant and young child nutrition.

38. Adequate *resources* – human, financial and organizational – will have to be identified and allocated to ensure the plan's timely successful implementation. Constructive dialogue and active collaboration with appropriate groups working for the protection, promotion and support of appropriate feeding practices will be particularly important in this connection. Support for epidemiological and operational research is also a crucial component.

Other concerned parties

39. Identifying specific responsibilities within society – crucial complementary and mutually reinforcing roles – for protecting, promoting and supporting appropriate feeding practices is something of a new departure. Groups that have an important role in advocating the rights of women and children and in creating a supportive environment on their behalf can work singly, together and with governments and international organizations to improve the situation by helping to remove both cultural and practical barriers to appropriate infant and young child feeding practices.

Health professional bodies

40. Health professional bodies, which include medical faculties, schools of public health, public and private institutions for training health workers (including midwives, nurses, nutritionists and dietitians), and professional associations, should have the following main responsibilities towards their students or membership:

- ensuring that basic education and training for all health workers cover lactation physiology, exclusive and continued breastfeeding, complementary feeding, feeding in difficult circumstances, meeting the nutritional needs of infants who have to be fed on breast-milk substitutes, and the International Code of Marketing of Breast-milk Substitutes and the legislation and other measures adopted to give effect to it and to subsequent relevant Health Assembly resolutions;

- training in how to provide skilled support for exclusive and continued breastfeeding, and appropriate complementary feeding in all neonatal, paediatric, reproductive health, nutritional and community health services;

- promoting achievement and maintenance of "baby-friendly" status by maternity hospitals, wards and clinics, consistent with the "Ten steps to successful breastfeeding"[1] and the principle of not accepting free or low-cost supplies of breast-milk substitutes, feeding bottles and teats;

- observing, in their entirety, their responsibilities under the International Code of Marketing of Breast-milk Substitutes and subsequent relevant Health Assembly resolutions, and national measures adopted to give effect to both;

- encouraging the establishment and recognition of community support groups and referring mothers to them.

Nongovernmental organizations including community-based support groups

41. The aims and objectives of a wide variety of nongovernmental organizations operating locally, nationally and internationally include promoting the adequate food and nutrition needs of young children and families. For example, charitable and religious organizations, consumer associations, mother-to-mother support groups, family clubs, and child-care cooperatives all have multiple opportunities to contribute to the implementation of this strategy through, for example:

- providing their members accurate, up-to-date information about infant and young child feeding;

- integrating skilled support for infant and young child feeding in community-based interventions and ensuring effective linkages with the health care system;

---

[1] *Protecting, promoting and supporting breastfeeding: the special role of maternity services.* A joint WHO/UNICEF statement. Geneva, WHO, 1989.

- contributing to the creation of mother- and child-friendly communities and workplaces that routinely support appropriate infant and young child feeding;

- working for full implementation of the principles and aim of the International Code of Marketing of Breast-milk Substitutes and subsequent relevant Health Assembly resolutions.

42. Parents and other caregivers are most directly responsible for feeding children. Ever keen to ensure that they have accurate information to make appropriate feeding choices, parents nevertheless are limited by their immediate environment. Since they may have only infrequent contact with the health care system during a child's first two years of life, it is not unusual for caregivers to be more influenced by community attitudes than by the advice of health workers.

43. Additional sources of information and support are found in a variety of formal and informal groups, including breastfeeding-support and child-care networks, clubs and religious associations. Community-based support, including that provided by other mothers, lay and peer breastfeeding counsellors and certified lactation consultants, can effectively enable women to feed their children appropriately. Most communities have self-help traditions that could readily serve as a base for building or expanding suitable support systems to help families in this regard.

Commercial enterprises

44. Manufacturers and distributors of industrially processed foods intended for infants and young children also have a constructive role to play in achieving the aim of this strategy. They should ensure that processed food products for infants and children, when sold, meet applicable Codex Alimentarius standards and the Codex Code of Hygienic Practice for Foods for Infants and Children. In addition, all manufacturers and distributors of products within the scope of the International Code of Marketing of Breast-milk Substitutes, including feeding bottles and teats, are responsible for monitoring their marketing practices according to the principles and aim of the Code. They should ensure that their conduct at every level conforms to the Code, subsequent relevant Health Assembly resolu-

tions, and national measures that have been adopted to give effect to both.

The social partners

45. *Employers* should ensure that maternity entitlements of all women in paid employment are met, including breastfeeding breaks or other workplace arrangements – for example facilities for expressing and storing breast milk for later feeding by a caregiver – in order to facilitate breast-milk feeding once paid maternity leave is over. *Trade unions* have a direct role in negotiating adequate maternity entitlements and security of employment for women of reproductive age (see paragraphs 28 and 34).

Other groups

46. Many other components of society have potentially influential roles in promoting good feeding practices. These elements include:

- *education authorities*, which help to shape the attitudes of children and adolescents about infant and young child feeding – accurate information should be provided through schools and other educational channels to promote greater awareness and positive perceptions;

- *mass media*, which influence popular attitudes towards parenting, child care and products within the scope of the International Code of Marketing of Breast-milk Substitutes – their information on the subject and, just as important, the way they portray parenting, childcare and products should be accurate, up to date, objective, and consistent with the Code's principles and aim;

- *child-care facilities*, which permit working mothers to care for their infants and young children, should support and facilitate continued breastfeeding and breast-milk feeding.

International organizations

47. International organizations, including global and regional lending institutions, should place infant and young child feeding high on the global public health agenda in recognition of its central significance for realizing the rights of children and women; they should

serve as advocates for increased human, financial and institutional resources for the universal implementation of this strategy; and, to the extent possible, they should provide additional resources for this purpose.

48. Specific contributions of international organizations to facilitate the work of governments include the following:

Developing norms and standards

- developing evidence-based guidelines to facilitate achievement of the strategy's operational targets;

- supporting epidemiological and operational research;

- promoting the consistent use of common global indicators for monitoring and evaluating child-feeding trends;

- developing new indicators, for example concerning adequate complementary feeding;

- improving the quality and availability of sex-disaggregated global, regional and national data;

Supporting national capacity-building

- sensitizing and training health policy-makers and health service administrators;

- improving health worker skills in support of optimal infant and young child feeding;

- revising related pre-service curricula for doctors, nurses, midwives, nutritionists, dietitians, auxiliary health workers and other groups as necessary;

- planning and monitoring the Baby-friendly Hospital Initiative and expanding it beyond the maternity-care setting;

- helping to ensure sufficient resources for this purpose, especially in highly indebted countries;

Supporting policy development and promotion

- supporting social-mobilization activities, for example using the mass media to promote appropriate infant feeding practices and educating media representatives;

- advocating ratification of ILO Maternity Protection Convention 2000 No. 183 and application of Recommendation 2000 No. 191, including for women in atypical forms of dependent work;

- urging implementation of the International Code of Marketing of Breast-milk Substitutes and subsequent relevant Health Assembly resolutions, and providing related technical support on request;

- ensuring that all Codex Alimentarius standards and related texts dealing with foods for infants and young children give full consideration to WHO policy concerning appropriate marketing and distribution, recommended age of use, and safe preparation and feeding, including as reflected in the International Code of Marketing of Breast-milk Substitutes and subsequent relevant Health Assembly resolutions;

- ensuring that the International Code of Marketing of Breast-milk Substitutes and subsequent relevant Health Assembly resolutions are given full consideration in trade policies and negotiations;

- supporting research on marketing practices and the International Code.

Conclusion

49. This strategy describes essential interventions to protect, promote and support appropriate infant and young child feeding. It focuses on the importance of investing in this crucial area to ensure that children develop to their full potential, free from the adverse consequences of compromised nutritional status and preventable illnesses. It concentrates on the roles of critical partners – governments, international organizations and other concerned parties – and assigns specific responsibilities for each to ensure that the sum of their collective action will contribute to the full attainment of the strategy's aim and objectives. It builds on existing approaches, extended where necessary, and provides a framework for linking synergistically the contributions of multiple programme areas, including nutrition, child health and development, and maternal and reproductive health. The strategy now needs to be translated into action.

50. There is convincing evidence from around the world that governments, with the support of the international community and other concerned parties, are taking seriously their commitments to protect and promote the health and nutritional well-being of infants, young children, and pregnant and lactating women.[1] One of the enduring tangible results of the International Conference on Nutrition, namely the World Declaration on Nutrition, offers a challenging vision of a world transformed. Meanwhile, its Plan of Action for Nutrition charts a credible course for achieving this transformation.[2]

51. In the decade since its adoption, 159 Member States (83%) have demonstrated their determination to act by preparing or strengthening their national nutrition policies and plans. More than half (59%) have included specific strategies to improve infant and young child feeding practices. This encouraging result needs to be consolidated, and expanded to include *all* Member States, even as it is reviewed and updated to ensure that it takes full account of the present comprehensive agenda. Clearly, however, much more is required if the aim and objectives of this strategy – and present and future feeding challenges – are to be met.

52. This global strategy provides governments and society's other main agents with both a valuable opportunity and a practical instrument for rededicating themselves, individually and collectively, to protecting, promoting and supporting safe and adequate feeding for infants and young children everywhere.

---

[1] Document A55/14.

[2] *World Declaration and Plan of Action for Nutrition.* International Conference on Nutrition, Rome, FAO and WHO, 1992.

ANNEX
Resolution WHA55.25 Infant and young child nutrition

The Fifty-fifth World Health Assembly,

Having considered the draft global strategy for infant and young-child feeding;

Deeply concerned about the vast numbers of infants and young children who are still inappropriately fed and whose nutritional status, growth and development, health and very survival are thereby compromised;

Conscious that every year as much as 55% of infant deaths from diarrhoeal disease and acute respiratory infections may be the result of inappropriate feeding practices, that less than 35% of infants worldwide are exclusively breastfed for even the first four months of life, and that complementary feeding practices are frequently ill-timed, inappropriate and unsafe;

Alarmed at the degree to which inappropriate infant and young-child feeding practices contribute to the global burden of disease, including malnutrition and its consequences such as blindness and mortality due to vitamin A deficiency, impaired psychomotor development due to iron deficiency and anaemia, irreversible brain damage as a consequence of iodine deficiency, the massive impact on morbidity and mortality of protein-energy malnutrition, and the later-life consequences of childhood obesity;

Recognizing that infant and young-child mortality can be reduced through improved nutritional status of women of reproductive age, especially during pregnancy, and by exclusive breastfeeding for the first six months of life, and with nutritionally adequate and safe complementary feeding through introduction of safe and adequate amounts of indigenous foodstuffs and local foods while breastfeeding continues up to the age of two years or beyond;

Mindful of the challenges posed by the ever-increasing number of people affected by major emergencies, the HIV/AIDS pandemic, and the complexities of modern lifestyles coupled with continued promulgation of inconsistent messages about infant and young-child feeding;

Aware that inappropriate feeding practices and their consequences are major obstacles to sustainable socioeconomic development and poverty reduction;

Reaffirming that mothers and babies form an inseparable biological and social unit, and that the health and nutrition of one cannot be divorced from the health and nutrition of the other;

Recalling the Health Assembly's endorsement, in their entirety, of the statement and recommendations made by the joint WHO/UNICEF Meeting on Infant and Young Child Feeding (1979) (resolution WHA33.32); its adoption of the International Code of Marketing of Breast-milk Substitutes (resolution WHA34.22), in which it stressed that adoption of and adherence to the Code were a minimum requirement; its welcoming of the Innocenti Declaration on the Protection, Promotion and Support of Breastfeeding as a basis for international health policy and action (resolution WHA44.33); its urging encouragement and support for all public and private health facilities providing maternity services so that they become "baby-friendly" (resolution WHA45.34); its urging ratification and implementation of the Convention on the Rights of the Child as a vehicle for family health development (resolution WHA46.27); and its endorsement, in their entirety, of the World Declaration and Plan of Action for Nutrition adopted by the International Conference on Nutrition (Rome, 1992) (resolution WHA46.7);

Recalling also resolutions WHA35.26, WHA37.30, WHA39.28, WHA41.11, WHA43.3, WHA45.34, WHA46.7, WHA47.5, WHA49.15 and WHA54.2 on infant and young-child nutrition, appropriate feeding practices and related questions;

Recognizing the need for comprehensive national policies on infant and young-child feeding, including guidelines on ensuring appropriate feeding of infants and young children in exceptionally difficult circumstances;

Convinced that it is time for governments to renew their commitment to protecting and promoting the optimal feeding of infants and young children,

1. ENDORSES the global strategy for infant and young-child feeding;

2. EXHORTS Member States, as a matter of urgency:

    (1) to adopt and implement the global strategy, taking into account national circumstances, while respecting positive local traditions and values, as part of their overall nutrition and child-health policies and programmes, in order to ensure optimal feeding for all infants and young children, and to reduce the risks associated with obesity and other forms of malnutrition;

    (2) to strengthen existing, or establish new, structures for implementing the global strategy through the health and other concerned sectors, for monitoring and evaluating its effectiveness, and for guiding resource investment and management to improve infant and young-child feeding;

    (3) to define for this purpose, consistent with national circumstances:

       (a) national goals and objectives,

       (b) a realistic timeline for their achievement,

       (c) measurable process and output indicators that will permit accurate monitoring and evaluation of action taken and a rapid response to identified needs;

    (4) to ensure that the introduction of micronutrient interventions and the marketing of nutritional supplements do not replace, or undermine support for the sustainable practice of, exclusive breast-feeding and optimal complementary feeding;

    (5) to mobilize social and economic resources within society and to engage them actively in implementing the global strategy and in achieving its aims and objectives in the spirit of resolution WHA49.15;

3. CALLS UPON other international organizations and bodies, in particular ILO, FAO, UNICEF, UNHCR, UNFPA and UNAIDS, to give high priority, within their respective mandates and programmes and consistent with guidelines on conflict of interest, to provision of support to governments in implementing this global strategy, and invites donors to provide adequate funding for the necessary measures;

4. REQUESTS the Codex Alimentarius Commission to continue to give full consideration, within the framework of its operational mandate, to action it might take to improve the quality standards of processed foods for infants and young children and to promote their safe and proper use at an appropriate age, including through adequate labelling, consistent with the policy of WHO, in particular the International Code of Marketing of Breast-milk Substitutes, resolution WHA54.2, and other relevant resolutions of the Health Assembly;

5. REQUESTS the Director-General:

(1) to provide support to Member States, on request, in implementing this strategy, and in monitoring and evaluating its impact;

(2) to continue, in the light of the scale and frequency of major emergencies worldwide, to generate specific information and develop training materials aimed at ensuring that the feeding requirements of infants and young children in exceptionally difficult circumstances are met;

(3) to strengthen international cooperation with other organizations of the United Nations system and bilateral development agencies in promoting appropriate infant and young-child feeding;

(4) to promote continued cooperation with and among all parties concerned with implementing the global strategy.

Endorsement of the UNICEF Executive Board

The second regular session of the UNICEF Executive Board
17 September 2002

2002/12. Global strategy on infant and young child feeding

The Executive Board

Endorses the global strategy for infant and young child feeding, as presented in the report on *Infant and young child nutrition* (A55/15 of 16 April 2002) and as endorsed by the Fifty-fifth World Health Assembly in its resolution WHA55.25 of 18 May 2002.